DK *Natural Care Library*
GARLIC

IMMUNITY BOOSTER & HEART HELPER

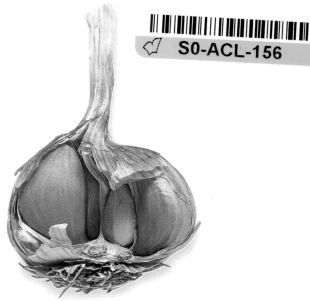

By STEPHANIE PEDERSEN

DORLING KINDERSLEY PUBLISHING, INC.
www.dk.com

CONTENTS

Herbal History 4

What is Garlic? 6

Science Talk 8

Rethinking Medication 10

Common Side Effects 12

Precautions 13

Formula Guide 14

Conditions and Doses 16

    Cardiovascular Conditions 16

    Cancer 22

    Common Colds, Influenza, and Other Infectious Diseases 24

    Diabetes 32

    Fatigue and Stress 34

    Intestinal Parasites 36

Conditions and Doses

Skin Conditions	38
Grow It Yourself	44
Do-It-Yourself Remedies	46
Herb Glossary	50
Herbal Terms	58
Herbal Organizations	60
Growing Herbs	61
Index	62

HERBAL HISTORY

Long before over-the-counter medications and prescription drugs came on the scene, herbs proved to be powerful healers. Every culture on earth has used herbal medicine. In fact, herbal usage is older than recorded history itself: Herbal preparations were found in the burial site of a Neanderthal man who lived over 60,000 years ago.

When it comes to herbal medicine, many healing systems are available and useful. Perhaps the best known are ayurveda, Chinese medicine, and Western herbalism. Ayurveda is a system of diagnosis and treatment that uses herbs in conjunction with breathing, meditation, and yoga. It has been practiced in India for more than 2,500 years. Ayurveda gets its name from the Sanskrit words *ayuh*, meaning "longevity," and *veda*, meaning "knowledge." Indeed, in ayurvedic healing, health can be achieved only after identifying a person's physical and mental characteristics (called *dosha*). Then the proper preventative or therapeutic remedies are prescribed to help an individual maintain doshic balance.

Chinese medicine is another healing system that uses herbs, in combination with acupressure, acupuncture, and qi gong. Sometimes called traditional Chinese medicine (TCM), this ancient system is thought to be rooted as far back as 2,800 BC in the time of emperor Sheng Nung. Known as China's patron saint of herbal medicine, Sheng Nung is credited among the first proponents of healing plants. Chinese medicine attempts to help the body correct energy imbalances. Therefore herbs are classified according to certain active characteristics, such as heating, cooling, moisturizing, or drying, and prescribed according to how they influence the activity of various organ systems.

Many herbal practitioners believe that Western herbalism can trace its roots to the ancient Sumerians, who—according to a medicinal recipe dating from 3000 BC—boasted a refined knowledge of herbal medicine. Records from subsequent cultures, such as the Assyrians, Egyptians, Israelites, Greeks, and Romans, show similar herbal healing systems. But these peoples weren't the only ones using beneficial plants. The Celts, Gauls, Scandinavians, and other early European tribes also healed with herbs. In fact, it was their knowledge, melded with the medicine brought by invading Moors and Romans, that formed the foundation for Western herbalism. Simply put, this foundation formed a comprehensive system wherein herbs were grouped according to how they affected both the body and specific body systems.

Western herbalism was refined further when Europeans traveled to the New World. Once here, the Europeans fused their medical knowledge with that of the Native Americans. Herbal know-how became an important part of early American habits, so that wellness remedies were handed down from mothers to daughters to granddaughters, and medicinal plants were grown in home gardens. Physicians from the 1600s, 1700s, 1800s, and early 1900s commonly used plants, such as arnica, echinacea, and garlic to heal patients. Herbs were listed as medicine in official publications such as the *United States Pharmacopoeia* (the definitive American listing) and the *National Formulary* (the pharmacist's handbook). With the creation of synthetic medications in the 1930s, herbal medicine began to wane.

Fortunately, Europeans and Asians never gave up their herbal remedies. Instead, they used them to complement synthetic medications. Their successes—combined with the desire of many Americans for alternatives to the high price tags and unforgiving side effects of synthetic drugs—have kept the world moving forward on a healthier herbal path.

What is Garlic?

Garlic is everywhere. Walk the aisles of any health food store and you can't miss it: garlic in capsules, liquid extracts, tinctures, and more. Yet garlic is no medicinal newcomer—the herb boasts a long, distinguished history as an anthelmintic, antibiotic, antiviral, astringent, and immune-system stimulant. Cuneiform tablets from 3000 BC have shown that Sumerians and Assyrians used garlic to strengthen the body and treat infectious fevers, diarrhea, swollen joints, and sprains. Sanskrit records dating from the same period show that in India people were using garlic for coughs, skin problems, hemorrhoids, worms, and leprosy. The Egyptian Ebers Codes, circa 1550 BC, gives 22 uses for garlic, including animal and insect bites, heart conditions, and worms; ancient Chinese, Greek, Israelite and Roman healers used garlic for many of the same ailments. Of special interest to the English-speaking world are the early Anglo-Saxons, who used an herb called garleac for poisoning and snake bites. In old English, the name meant "spear-leek" and referred to the shape of garlic's spearlike stem.

Today, garlic may be best-known as an infection fighter that is especially helpful in boosting immune system function, inhibiting bacteria, and suppressing viruses. Garlic contains a volatile oil comprised of sulfur-containing compounds: ajoene, alliin (which converts into allicin when garlic is crushed or injured in any way), diallyl disulfide, diallyl trisulfide, and others. These volatile compounds are responsible for most of garlic's pharmacological properties. Other elements include enzymes, glucosinolates, protein, selenium, S-methyl-L-cysteine sulfoxide, and vitamins.

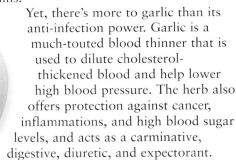

Yet, there's more to garlic than its anti-infection power. Garlic is a much-touted blood thinner that is used to dilute cholesterol-thickened blood and help lower high blood pressure. The herb also offers protection against cancer, inflammations, and high blood sugar levels, and acts as a carminative, digestive, diuretic, and expectorant.

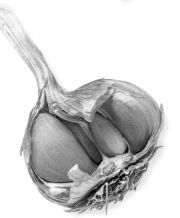

IN OTHER WORDS
Like many herbs, Garlic is known by several names. Here are a few of them:

* ☆ **Allium Sativum**
* ☆ **Camphor of the Poor**
* ☆ **Nectar of the Gods**
* ☆ **Maindenhair Tree**
* ☆ **Poor Man's Treacle**
* ☆ **Rustic Treacle**
* ☆ **Stinking Rose**

SCIENCE TALK

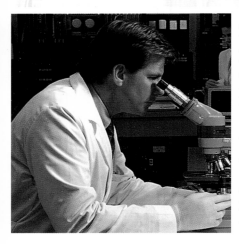

MEDICINE WORLDWIDE

The National Institutes of Health, in Bethesda, MD, estimate that only 10 to 30 percent of the health care worldwide is allopathic, or "Western." The rest of the world's medical care is what Americans would call "alternative," including ayurveda, energy healing, herbalism, homeopathy and traditional Chinese medicine.

CELEBRATING GERMAN KNOW-HOW

Perhaps no other country in the Western world has done more than Germany to further the cause of herbal medicine. What's the country's secret? Commission E, a review board of respected pharmacologists, physicians and scientists. The board was established in 1978, and members spent the first 15 years researching more than 300 age-old herbal remedies for usages, recommended dosages, preparations and side effects. Then, in 1980, the German government upped the medical ante, creating a mandate requiring all new herbal remedies sold in pharmacies to meet the same criteria as over-the-counter drugs. To comply, researchers performed thousands of rigorous clinical trials, resulting in a deep well of knowledge used by doctors open to herbs worldwide.

DO YOU HAVE A CONTRAINDICATION?

Before taking any herb, it's important to ask your physician whether you have any contraindications. What does contraindication mean? It's a common medical term that refers to a symptom or condition that makes a particular treatment inadvisable. For example, when it comes to garlic, an anticlotting blood condition is a contraindication. Why? Adding the blood-thinning powers of garlic to this mix can create an even greater health hazard.

Before taking any herb, ask yourself the following questions:

✔ Have I done any background research on the herb?

✔ What condition am I taking this herb for?

✔ Am I taking other medications or herbs that may affect the herb's functioning?

✔ Do I have any pre-existing condition that is contraindicated?

✔ Am I pregnant, trying to conceive or nursing?

✔ Have I spoken to my physician, a naturopathic doctor or an herbalist before taking herb?

✔ Do I know the proper dosages for the herb?

RETHINKING MEDICATION

ANTIBIOTICS: ARE THEY ESSENTIAL?

A recent report published in the *Journal of the American Medical Association* stated that even though antibiotics provide little help for colds, upper respiratory tract infections and bronchitis, doctors still prescribe antibiotics for these conditions. Why? In part, because patients expect their doctors to give them some kind of medication, and many physicians find it easier to oblige than take time out to explain how antibiotics do and don't work. Americans are so enamored of antibiotics that doctors write over 12 million antibiotic prescriptions annually. To learn more about the dangers of antibiotic abuse, contact the Centers For Disease Control and Prevention, 404-332-4555.

PENICILLIN BY THE POUND

Since penicillin's debut in 1941, antibiotic production has shot up from 2 million pounds in 1954 to more than 50 million pounds in 1997. Where is all this medication going? Half of the antibiotics produced annually are prescribed for people; the rest are mixed into livestock feed and used as fertilizers for agricultural crops. The downside to this free-flowing penicillin? New, strong, antibiotic-resistant strains of bacteria.

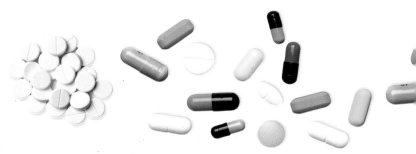

WAIT! BEFORE YOU TAKE THAT PILL . . .
Before asking your doctor for an antibiotic, ask yourself the
following questions:

✔ Is my condition caused by bacteria? If not, antibiotics
  will not work.

✔ Are antibiotics necessary for recovery? If the infection
  will go away on its own, consider forgoing antibiotics.

✔ Are there alternatives to antibiotics? If herbal or other
  natural remedies can fight off the infection, consider
  using one or more of them.

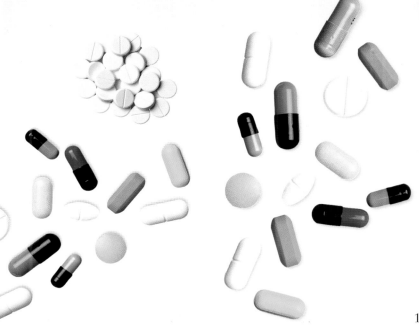

COMMON SIDE EFFECTS

Many medicinal herbs cause mild side effects. Here's what a small number of garlic-users experience:

☆ Diarrhea
☆ Flatulence
☆ Flushed Face
☆ Gastric Irritation
☆ Headache
☆ Heartburn
☆ Insomnia
☆ Nausea
☆ Rapid Pulse
☆ Skin Irritation (with external applications)
☆ Vomiting

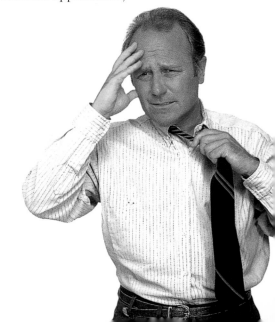

PRECAUTIONS

✖ When used in culinary amounts—two cloves minced and added to an eight-serving recipe of lasagna, and perhaps another clove whisked into a large batch of salad dressing—garlic is safe for everyone. It is only high medicinal doses of the herb that can cause trouble for certain individuals.

✖ Because garlic can thin the blood when taken in large amounts, individuals who are on blood-thinning medication or whose blood does not clot should talk with their physicians before taking medicinal doses of garlic.

✖ During and after surgery, blood clotting is necessary to prevent bleeding complications. Thus, garlic's blood-thinning qualities make it hazardous in high doses to individuals who are awaiting surgery. If you have a surgery scheduled, refrain from taking garlic for two weeks beforehand.

✖ When used externally, the volatile oils in garlic can cause irritation and sometimes blistering in individuals with sensitive skin.

✖ Medicinal doses of garlic slightly lower blood sugar levels. Hypoglycemics should consult their physicians before taking large amounts of garlic.

✖ If you are pregnant, nursing, trying to conceive, or are taking any type of medication, please consult your physician before using garlic.

FORMULA GUIDE

Capsules, extracts, teas, tinctures—what do they all mean?
For the uninitiated, we offer this guide to herbal formulas:

☆ **Capsules.** The medicinal part of the herb is freeze-dried, pulverized, and packed into gelatin capsules. Garlic capsules usually contain anywhere from 300 mg to 350 mg of herb powder; occasionally the dried herb is reinforced with concentrated extracts. In the case of garlic, some companies even manufacture capsules containing up to 1500 mg of garlic oil.

☆ **Herb, Dried.** The flowers, leaves, stems, and/or roots of many herbs are often available dried at health food stores and herbal pharmacies. While these are most commonly made into homemade teas, they can also be used to make decoctions, infused oils, sachets, and more.

☆ **Herb, Fresh.** Herbs that are used in both culinary and medicinal ways (such as dill, garlic, and parsley) are most often found fresh. These can be made into homemade extract, juice, infused oil, tea, and more.

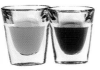

☆ **Juices.** The extracted juice from fresh herbs can be found mixed with commercially prepared fruit or vegetable juices.

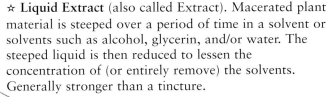

☆ **Liquid Extract** (also called Extract). Macerated plant material is steeped over a period of time in a solvent or solvents such as alcohol, glycerin, and/or water. The steeped liquid is then reduced to lessen the concentration of (or entirely remove) the solvents. Generally stronger than a tincture.

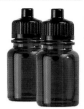

☆ **Oil, Essential** (also called Oil). Essential oils are the volatile oily components of herbs. They are found in tiny glands located in the flowers, leaves, roots, and/or bark and are mechanically or chemically extracted. Essential oil is prescribed almost exclusively for external use.

☆ **Oil, Infused.** Made by steeping fresh or dried herbs in an edible oil. After a period of time, the herbs are removed and the oil used internally or externally. Not as potent as essential oil.

☆ **Ointments.** Dried or fresh herbs are steeped in a base of oils and emulsifiers (such as beeswax, petroleum jelly, or soft paraffin wax). After a period of time, the herbs are removed and the ointment packaged. For external use only.

☆ **Syrups.** Syrups are usually a combination of herbal extracts and a sweetener, such as honey or sugar. Generally used for colds, flu, and sore throats.

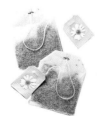

☆ **Teas/Infusions.** The words "tea" and "infusion" are often used interchangeably in herbal healing. While commercial herbal tea bags are available, herbal tea can also be made with loose dried or fresh herbs.

☆ **Tinctures.** Plant material is soaked in alcohol. The saturated plant material is then pressed. Liquid from this pressing may be diluted with water and packaged—usually in small dropper bottles.

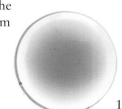

Natural Care

CONDITIONS AND DOSES

CORONARY ARTERY DISEASE

❑ **Symptoms:** Coronary artery disease accounts for about one in two American deaths each year. The disease progresses slowly over the course of years and even decades, but its impact can be instantaneous: In nearly one-third of all cases, death occurs without any previous warning of disease. Indeed, some people have no symptoms, while others may experience chest pain, constriction or a sense of heaviness in the chest, fatigue, pallor, shortness of breath, swelling in the ankles, and/or weakness. Coronary artery disease occurs when cholesterol deposits build up on coronary artery walls. These special blood vessels provide oxygen and nutrients to the muscles of the heart. Yet when they are unable to deliver adequate blood flow, the heart muscle begins to weaken, leading to angina (chest pain), congestive heart failure, and heart attack. When it comes to causes, a high-fat diet is most often implicated, although heredity, stress, inactivity, smoking, and alcoholism are also culprits.

❑ **How Garlic Can Help:** Several studies have shown that garlic combats coronary artery disease in two ways. The alliin and diallyl sulfides in garlic are powerful antioxidants that help kill artery-damaging free radicals created by cholesterol deposits. Allicin keeps blood platelets from becoming sticky and thick; thin blood can more easily pass through blocked arteries.

❏ **Dosages:** If you are currently being treated for coronary artery disease, do not take large amounts of garlic without first consulting your cardiologist. If given the go-ahead, take at least 4 grams of fresh, raw garlic a day. This is the equivalent of one large garlic clove. Or take one 300-milligram capsule three times daily; or 5 grams of liquid extract three times daily; or 5 grams of tincture three times daily. Garlic can be taken indefinitely

WHAT TO LOOK FOR?

In the market for a garlic remedy, but you're not sure how to choose one? Your best bet may be your supermarket's produce aisle. Garlic contains a volatile oil composed of sulfur-containing compounds: ajoene, alliin (which converts into allicin when garlic is crushed or injured in any way), diallyl disulfide, diallyl trisulfide, and others. These volatile compounds are responsible for most of garlic's pharmacological properties. And because many of these compounds are inactivated by heat and processing, raw garlic contains the greatest percentage of the herb's medicinal benefits.

That said, what if you'd rather take your garlic in a capsule, extract, tincture, or some other form? To ensure that you get the most potent—and beneficial—medicine available, look for products containing at least 10 milligrams of alliin or a total allicin potential of 4,000 micrograms. This amount is equal to approximately one clove of fresh garlic.

CONDITIONS AND DOSES

HIGH BLOOD CHOLESTEROL

❒ **Symptoms:** High blood cholesterol refers to high levels of fat in the blood. Blame the condition on a fatty diet, heredity, alcoholism, smoking, sedentary lifestyle, or a combination thereof—whatever the cause, the condition is dangerous. Gummy in texture, fat thickens blood and gets stuck on artery walls, impeding adequate blood flow to the heart and brain and thus increasing one's risk of coronary artery disease, heart attack, and stroke. Symptoms can include chest pain, lethargy, pallor, and shortness of breath. However, the condition is often asymptomatic; many individuals learn they have high cholesterol only after a routine blood test.

❒ **How Garlic Can Help:** Garlic is one of many complementary measures that lower high blood cholesterol levels. Important steps include adopting a low-fat vegetarian or near-vegetarian diet, quitting cigarettes, and exercising regularly. Several American and European studies have found that garlic reduces total serum cholesterol and triglyceride levels, as well as thinning fat-thickened blood.

❒ **Dosages:** If you are currently being treated for high cholesterol, do not take large amounts of garlic without first consulting your cardiologist. If given the go-ahead, take at least 4 grams of fresh, raw garlic a day. This is the equivalent of one large garlic clove. Or, take one 300-mg capsule three times daily; or 5 grams of liquid extract three times daily; or 5 grams of tincture three times daily. Garlic can be taken indefinitely.

LIMIT CHEMICAL EXPOSURE

It's nearly impossible to avoid all chemical toxins in today's world. There's ammonia in cleaning products, chlorine in the water, lead in old paint and pipes, dibromochloropropane in pesticides, carbon monoxide from auto exhaust, and toluene, trichloroethylene, and formaldehyde from printers, photocopiers, and fax machines. Many of these toxins have been linked to allergies, breathing problems, cancer, headaches, infertility, lethargy, lung conditions, reduced attention span, and violence. Ideas for lessening toxins include using environmentally sound dry cleaning, drinking filtered water, purchasing (or making) natural cleansers, limiting the amount of driving you do, and adding a few chemical-filtering plants such as dracaena, chrysanthemum, and weeping fig (ficus) to your home.

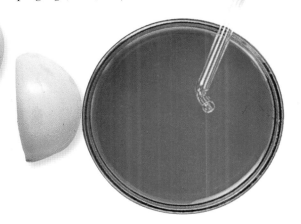

CONDITIONS AND DOSES

HYPERTENSION

❏ **Symptoms:** Hypertension, more commonly known as high blood pressure, is a condition in which blood travels through the arteries at higher-than-normal pressure. This increased blood flow literally wears out the blood vessels, heart, and kidneys—and can lead to premature death. What causes hypertension? Cigarettes, alcohol, some medications, and certain illnesses can elevate blood pressure—but by far the most common cause of hypertension is clogged arteries from a high-fat diet. When blood vessels are blocked with fatty deposits, the heart must work harder to move the same amount of blood through them. This in turn increases the pressure at which the blood is pumped. Unfortunately, hypertension is symptomless, leaving many individuals unaware that they even suffer from the condition—until it's too late.

❏ **How Garlic Can Help:** Garlic helps treat hypertension in two ways: First, it inhibits coagulation, so blood doesn't clog on cholesterol deposits as it moves through the arteries. Secondly, studies have shown that garlic significantly decreases the pressure in which blood travels through the arteries.

❏ **Dosages:** If you are currently being treated for hypertension, do not take large amounts of garlic without first consulting your cardiologist. If given the go-ahead, take at least 4 grams of fresh, raw garlic a day. This is the equivalent of one large garlic clove. Or, take one 300-mg capsule three times daily; or 5 grams of liquid extract three times daily; or 5 grams of tincture three times daily. Garlic can be taken indefinitely.

THEY DON'T CALL IT THE STINKING ROSE FOR NOTHING!

Who doesn't love garlic? It adds life to any dish while providing a range of health benefits. But—and this is a big "but," as anyone who's been cornered by someone with garlic breath can tell you—garlic can really stink up a person's breath. Switching to garlic capsules can lessen garlic breath, but it won't eliminate it entirely. That's because highly-odiferous sulfurous constituents are what give garlic and garlic products their benefits. Fortunately, there's no need to choose between the health benefits of garlic and a happy social life. Here are three simple ways to wipe out the dreaded "garlic breath":

☆ Eat 1 or 2 tablespoons of raw parsley after consuming garlic or garlic products.

☆ Munch on 2 teaspoons of fennel seeds after consuming garlic or garlic products.

☆ Chew 2 or 3 cardamom seeds after consuming garlic or garlic products.

CONDITIONS AND DOSES

CANCER

❏ **Symptoms:** Cancer occurs when cells begin growing abnormally, forming malignant tumors. These malignant tumors can appear in the breast, the bones, the throat, the brain, the stomach—actually, in almost any area of the body. But why do cells begin acting strange in the first place? It's believed that exposure to carcinogens causes body cells to mutate. Common carcinogens include cigarette smoke, fatty foods, industrial chemicals, insecticides, nuclear radiation, pesticides used on food, polluted air, and ultraviolet (UV) light. While cancer symptoms vary widely depending on what part of the body is affected, general signs include blood in the urine or stool, fatigue, hoarseness, indigestion, nagging cough, sores that do not heal, thickening somewhere in the body, and unexplained weight loss.

❏ **How Garlic Can Help:** Garlic has been used as a cancer preventative and treatment as far back as the fourth century BC when Hippocrates recommended the herb. And modern medicine backs him up. In animal studies, several components of garlic— ajoene, allicin, diallyl disulfide, diallyl sulfide, diallyl trisulfide, and selenium—boosted laboratory animals' resistance to cancer-causing chemicals and radiation and enhanced the animals' ability to resist implanted tumors. Furthermore, several large epidemiological studies have shown that individuals who eat some amount of fresh garlic daily have significantly lower cancer rates than individuals who do not consume garlic regularly.

❏ **Dosages:** Garlic has traditionally been used as a cancer preventative. The dosage is 4 grams of fresh, raw garlic a day. This is the equivalent of one large garlic clove. Or, take one 300 mg capsule three times daily; or 5 grams of liquid extract, three times daily; or 5 grams of tincture three times daily. Garlic can be taken indefinitely. Before using garlic to treat established cancer, consult your physician. The recommended dose is the same as above.

CANCER TREATMENT COMPANION

When a person gets cancer, the normal course of action is to physically remove as much of the malignantcy as possible, then follow up with a course of chemotherapy and/or radiation therapy. Chemotherapy uses drugs or a mixture of drugs to prevent any remaining cancerous cells from spreading. Radiation therapy employs a controlled beam of high-dose radiation aimed at the cancer-stricken area in order to kill cancerous cells. There are downsides to these two types of therapy, including extreme nausea, digestive problems, gastric upset, hair loss, and greatly-lowered immune-system function. Fortunately, there is a measure of help. It's called garlic. In a Japanese study, garlic was given to a group of women who were undergoing both chemotherapy and radiation therapy. Not only did the patients who used garlic have fewer side effects than those who did not, 67 percent of the women taking garlic reported no side effects at all.

CONDITIONS AND DOSES

ACUTE BRONCHITIS

❏ **Symptoms:** Acute bronchitis is a common illness characterized by inflammation of the bronchi, the breathing tubes that lead to the lungs. Caused by the same virus responsible for the common cold, bronchitis is characterized by constriction of the chest, chest pain, coughing (often with yellowish sputum), difficulty breathing, fatigue, fever, and sore throat.

❏ **How Garlic Can Help:** Allicin and the other sulfur components of garlic inhibit viruses in the body and simultaneously stimulate the body's production of protective antibodies. Garlic also strengthens the immune system, making it both more powerful and more efficient.

❏ **Dosages:** At the very first sign of illness, immediately take at least 8 grams of fresh, raw garlic a day. This is the equivalent of two large garlic cloves. Or take two 300-mg capsules three times daily; or 10 grams of liquid extract, three times daily; or 10 grams of tincture, three times daily. Garlic can be taken indefinitely.

To ease the sore throat that often accompanies acute bronchitis, gargle with garlic tea or decoction up to three times daily. Continue garlic therapy until symptoms are gone.

Garlic can also be used as a preventative during cold and flu season: Take at least 4 grams of fresh, raw garlic a day. This is the equivalent of one large garlic clove. Or take one 300-mg capsule three times daily; or 5 grams of liquid extract three times daily; or 5 grams of tincture three times daily. Garlic can be taken indefinitely.

START MOVING

Exercise boosts mood, improves immune-system function, prevents obesity, and strengthens muscles—all of which make exercise important for maintaining health. Fortunately for those who are too busy or too out-of-shape for regular gym workouts, studies have shown that small, five-minute bursts of exercise throughout the day—raking leaves instead of hiring a neighborhood teen to do it, using stairs instead of the elevator, walking to the corner store rather than driving—contribute to disease prevention, mood improvement, and overall well-being.

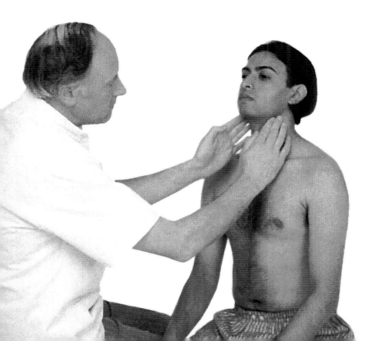

CONDITIONS AND DOSES

COLD

❏ **Symptoms:** Ever wonder why it's called the common cold? Because it is just that: common. In fact, it is estimated that healthy adults get an average of two colds per year. Most colds are caused by a rhinovirus, although in some instances bacteria can be to blame. Symptoms include coughing, nasal congestion, malaise, sneezing, sore throat, and watery eyes.

❏ **How Garlic Can Help:** Garlic is a classic cold remedy that has been used for centuries in Africa, the US, Asia, and Europe. According to several studies, it's an effective remedy, too. Garlic's strong antiviral ability deactivates a trespassing virus before it can cause illness. In addition, garlic strengthens the immune system, helping it to work more efficiently.

❏ **Dosages:** At the very first sign of illness, immediately take at least 8 grams of fresh, raw garlic a day. This is the equivalent of two large garlic cloves. Or, take two 300-mg capsules three times daily; or 10 grams of liquid extract three times daily; or 10 grams of tincture three times daily. Garlic can be taken indefinitely.

To ease the sore throat that often accompanies a cold, gargle with garlic tea or decoction up to three times daily. Continue garlic therapy until symptoms are gone.

Garlic can also be used as a preventative during cold and flu season: Take at least 4 grams of fresh, raw garlic a day. This is the equivalent of one large garlic clove. Or take one 300-mg capsule three times daily; or 5 grams of liquid extract three times daily; or 5 grams of tincture three times daily. Garlic can be taken indefinitely.

DID YOU KNOW?
Today, garlic may be best known as an infection fighter that is especially helpful in boosting immune system function, inhibiting bacteria, and suppressing viruses.

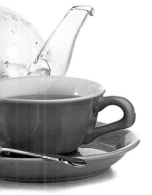

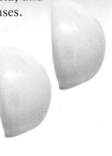

CONDITIONS AND DOSES

INFLUENZA

❐ **Symptoms:** Influenza, also known as the flu, is caused by a virus that is spread between people via infected droplets of air. Symptoms include coughing, fatigue, fever and chills, headache, muscular aches and pains, nasal congestion, sore throat, and weakness.

❐ **How Garlic Can Help:** Studies have shown that the sulfur-containing compounds in garlic block viral activity in the body and simultaneously strengthen the body's immune functioning.

❐ **Dosages:** At the very first sign of illness, immediately take at least 8 grams of fresh, raw garlic a day. This is the equivalent of two large garlic cloves. Or take two 300-mg capsules three times daily; or 10 grams of liquid extract three times daily; or 10 grams of tincture three times daily. Garlic can be taken indefinitely.

To ease the sore throat that often accompanies influenza, gargle with garlic tea or decoction up to three times daily. Continue garlic therapy until symptoms are gone.

Garlic can also be used as a preventative during cold and flu season: Take at least 4 grams of fresh, raw garlic a day. This is the equivalent of one large garlic clove. Or take one 300-mg capsule three times daily; or 5 grams of liquid extract three times daily; or 5 grams of tincture three times daily. Garlic can be taken indefinitely

SUSCEPTIBILITY TO INFECTIOUS ILLNESSES

❐ **Symptoms:** The average American gets two or three colds and one bout of flu each year. If you suffer from more than this, there's a chance you may have a poorly functioning immune system—which increases your susceptibility to infectious illnesses. Some people are born with weak immune systems, while others undermine their immunity with heavy drinking, poor diet, recreational drug use, smoking, or chronic stress.

❐ **How Garlic Can Help:** Garlic boasts immunity-boosting powers. American studies have found that diallyl trisulfide, a constituent of garlic, enhances the activity of macrophages, white blood cells that filter the blood and lymphatic system by destroying bacteria, viruses, and other waste matter. This, in turn, increases the body's defense system. Garlic also has broad antimicrobial powers, giving it the ability to destroy illness-causing bacteria, fungi, and viruses.

❐ **Dosages:** During cold and flu season, enjoy one to three cups of garlic tea daily. For stronger protection, take 4 grams of fresh, raw garlic a day. This is the equivalent of one large garlic cloves. Or take one 300-mg capsule three times daily; or 5 grams of liquid extract three times daily; or 5 grams of tincture three times daily. Garlic can be taken indefinitely.

To ease the sore throat that often accompanies acute respiratory infections, gargle with garlic tea or decoction up to three times daily. Continue garlic therapy until symptoms are gone. Garlic can be taken indefinitely.

CONDITIONS AND DOSES

MONONUCLEOSIS

❏ **Symptoms:** Mononucleosis is also called Epstein-Barr virus, after the Epstein-Barr herpes virus that causes the disease. It is transmitted when infectious saliva is spread through sneezing and coughing. Symptoms include abdominal pain, appetite loss, chest pain, coughing, difficulty breathing, fatigue, fever, general weakness, headache, sensitivity to light, sore throat, stiffness, and swollen lymph nodes.

❏ **How Garlic Can Help:** Several of garlic's constituents have been shown in clinical studies to kill viruses—including the herpes virus. In addition to deactivating the actual virus, garlic also strengthens the immune system. This is important, because a healthy immune system is better able to fight off any harmful organism that does slip into the body.

❏ **Dosages:** At the very first sign of illness, immediately take at least 8 grams of fresh, raw garlic a day. This is the equivalent of two large garlic cloves. Or take two 300-mg capsules three times daily; or 10 grams of liquid extract three times daily; or 10 grams of tincture three times daily. Garlic can be taken indefinitely.

To ease the sore throat that often accompanies mononucleosis, gargle with garlic tea or decoction up to three times daily. Continue garlic therapy until symptoms are gone.

Garlic can also be used as a preventative against viral infections such as mononucleosis: Take at least 4 grams of fresh, raw garlic a day. This is the equivalent of one large garlic clove. Or take one 300-mg capsule three times daily; or 5 grams of liquid extract three times daily; or 5 grams of tincture three times daily. Garlic can be taken indefinitely.

GO ORGANIC

When you use organic produce and prepared convenience foods made with organic ingredients, you're getting food that was grown without synthetic fertilizers, fungicides, and pesticides. Not only is this important for your own health—several of these substances have been linked to allergies, cancer, and lung conditions—but it's important for the environment. Many fertilizers, fungicides, and pesticides kill beneficial insects and animals, such as ants, butterflies, and frogs, as well as cause air pollution and contribute to the greenhouse effect. Pesticides also find their way into nearby wells, streams, and rivers. In fact, according to the Environmental Protection Agency, 40 percent of America's rivers, streams and lakes are not fit for fishing or swimming due to runoff of agricultural chemicals.

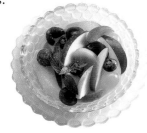

CONDITIONS AND DOSES

DIABETES

❐ **Symptoms:** To understand diabetes, it helps to know something about the pancreas. The organ—long and thin and situated behind the stomach—is responsible for regulating the body's use of glucose. To do so, the pancreas creates a number of chemicals, including insulin. When blood glucose levels begin to rise, it is insulin's job to prod muscle and fat cells to absorb whatever glucose they need for future activities; the liver stores any surplus. Yet some individuals either do not produce enough insulin (diabetes Type 1), or their bodies resist whatever insulin is produced (diabetes Type 2), and thus an outside source is required. Either way, the result is the same. Type 1, or juvenile-onset diabetes, typically affects children and young adults and is genetically linked. Type 2, or adult-onset diabetes, occurs in adults and is linked to obesity. Symptoms of both types include blurred vision, fatigue, frequent bladder infections, increased appetite, increased thirst, increased urination, nausea, skin infections, vaginitis, and vomiting. If not treated, diabetes Type 1 and Type 2 can cause blood vessel damage, gangrene, heart attack, kidney damage, nerve damage, stroke, and vision problems.

❐ **How Garlic Can Help:** Garlic is a popular diabetes treatment that can be used in tandem with diet and with traditional medication. Studies have shown that allicin and allyl propyl disulfide—two constituents of garlic—increase insulin levels in the body and lower blood sugar levels. Garlic has also been shown to lower the risk of coronary artery disease, a common complication of long-term diabetes.

❑ **Dosages:** Before taking garlic, speak with your physician about whether the herb is right for you. This is especially important if you are currently on medication for diabetes. The recommended dose is at least 4 grams of fresh, raw garlic a day. This is the equivalent of one large garlic clove. Or take one 300-mg capsule three times daily; or 5 grams of liquid extract three times daily; or 5 grams of tincture three times daily. Garlic can be taken indefinitely.

GARLIC'S SELF-PROTECTIVE INSTINCTS
Alliin is one of garlic's primary medicinal constituents. It's also a powerful antioxidant and detoxicant. However, should a garlic clove get bruised, banged, or cut, some of the alliin immediately converts to allicin. Why? The answer lies in self-defense—the plant's. A wound is an easy entry point for disease-causing bacteria, fungi, and viruses. Allicin, which boasts powerful antibiotic, antifungal, and antiviral properties, is the herb's safeguard against marauding microbes. Put another way: The same ingredient that shields garlic from disease is the very one that can help protect humans from illness.

CONDITIONS AND DOSES

FATIGUE

❑ **Symptoms:** Fatigue is a side effect of many medical and nonmedical conditions, including depression, illness, mental exertion, physical exertion, and stress. Signs of fatigue include mental and physical exhaustion, lethargy, sleepiness, and general weakness.

❑ **How Garlic Can Help:** It is not known exactly how garlic combats fatigue, but the herb has a long history as a tonic. In fact, records show that the laborers who built the Egyptian pyramids used garlic to fight fatigue. More modern accounts include a Japanese study that followed two groups of athletes—one that took garlic and one that took a placebo. For three weeks, all individuals performed three hours of highly rigorous exercise each day. At the end of the study, the garlic-takers experienced less physical fatigue, had faster physical and mental reflexes, and reported more energy than the placebo group.

❑ **Dosages:** During periodic times of fatigue, enjoy one to three cups of garlic tea daily. Garlic can also be used as a daily supplement to help combat long-term fatigue. However, before supplementing with garlic, speak with your physician about whether the herb is right for you. The dosage is 4 grams of fresh, raw garlic a day. This is the equivalent of one large garlic clove. Or take one 300-mg capsule three times daily; or 5 grams of liquid extract three times daily; or 5 grams of tincture three times daily. Garlic can be taken indefinitely.

STRESS

❐ **Symptoms:** Who doesn't experience periods of stress? Whether caused by increased demands at work, money worries, relationship woes, or something else entirely, stress prompts the body to release what are called stress hormones, such as epinephrine and cortisol. These hormones help increase blood flow to the muscles and prepare the body for a short period of extreme exertion. However, in times of ongoing anxiety, high levels of these hormones hang around in the body, causing changes in appetite, gastrointestinal upset, headaches, impaired concentration, irritability, muscle tension, sleeplessness, and teeth grinding.

❐ **How Garlic Can Help:** Several American and Japanese animal and human studies have found that garlic enhances the body's ability to cope with stress. Garlic lowers stress hormone levels in the body. Very simply put, the less of these hormones in the body, the weaker the body's physical response to stress. Garlic also strengthens immune-system function, which can be severely weakened by stress.

❐ **Dosages:** During periodic stressful times, enjoy one to three cups of garlic tea daily. Garlic can also be used as a daily supplement to help combat long-term stress. However, before supplementing with garlic, speak with your physician about whether the herb is right for you. Take at least 4 grams of fresh, raw garlic a day. This is the equivalent of one large garlic clove. Or take one 300-mg capsule three times daily; or 5 grams of liquid extract three times daily; or 5 grams of tincture three times daily. Garlic can be taken indefinitely.

CONDITIONS AND DOSES

INTESTINAL PARASITES

❏ **Symptoms:** There are a number of parasites that can affect the intestinal tract. These include ascarias, tapeworms, pinworms, and strongyles. These parasites typically live in infected animal tissue or water and can be transmitted to humans who ingest either infected meat or water. Symptoms can include anal itching, abdominal bloating, abdominal pain, anemia, diarrhea, dizziness, fatigue, headache, low-grade fever, malabsorption of food, muscle pain, muscle tenderness, nausea, and vomiting. Intestinal parasites are extremely rare in the United States and western Europe; most Americans and western Europeans who become infected with parasites do so while traveling outside their countries.

❏ **How Garlic Can Help:** Garlic enjoys a long-trusted history as an anti parasitic agent, having been used by early Assyrians, Egyptians, Greeks, Romans, and Sumerians for just that purpose. Though scientists don't know exactly how garlic kills and expels parasites from the body, several modern human studies have proven its effectiveness.

❑ **Dosages:** At the very first sign of illness, immediately take at least 8 grams of fresh, raw garlic a day; unfortunately, commercial garlic products are not as effective as garlic in its natural, raw state. Discontinue garlic therapy when parasites have been eradicated.

EAT A PLANT-BASED DIET
What do cancer, coronary artery disease, diabetes, digestive disorders, diverticulitis, gallstones, hemorrhoids, high blood pressure, and obesity, have in common? They all can be prevented or helped by a high-fiber plant-based diet. If you don't want to entirely rid your diet of lean beef, fish, lamb, pork, poultry, and other meats, limit yourself to two or three servings per week (yes, per week, not day), and be sure to get five or more servings of fruits and vegetables daily.

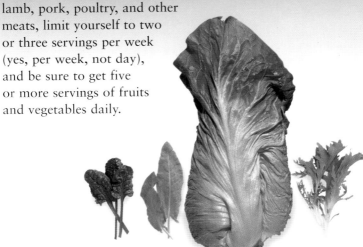

CONDITIONS AND DOSES

ACNE

❏ **Symptoms:** Acne is an inflammatory skin disorder. It occurs when hormones stimulate the overproduction of keratin and sebum, which in turn get caught in the skin's pores, causing blackheads. Often bacteria mixes with the excess keratin and sebum, resulting in infected whiteheads and cystlike pustules. While acne generally affects the face, it also occurs on the neck, chest, and back, and can be mild to severe.

❏ **How Garlic Can Help:** When used externally, garlic's strong antibacterial action kills pimple-causing bacteria on the skin. The herb's astringent action also helps eliminate excess sebum from the skin's surface.

❏ **Dosages:** Apply a garlic poultice or fomentation directly to whiteheads and pustules up to two times daily. As a preventative, fresh garlic tea or decoction can be used as a toner. Moisten a cotton ball or clean washcloth with tea or decoction and apply to the face immediately after cleansing.

EXTERNAL MATTERS

When used externally, garlic effectively eradicates bacteria, fungi, and viruses, from the skin's surface. However, individuals with sensitive skin may find that garlic is a little too powerful. Many sensitive individuals experience burning, itching, and inflammation, after topical applications of the herb. Even nonsensitive individuals should be careful about not over using garlic externally.

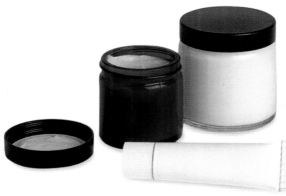

CONDITIONS AND DOSES

BOILS

❐ **Symptoms:** Boils generally occur in individuals with weak immune systems. Known medically as furuncles, boils are inflamed, pus-filled nodules that occur when the *staphylococcus aureus* bacteria infect a hair follicle. The bacteria then bore into the skin's deeper layers. The result is localized itching, pain, and redness. A mild fever and swollen lymph glands may also occur.

❐ **How Garlic Can Help:** Because boils are contagious, it is important to have a physician lance the boil and remove the infectious pus. Used externally, garlic is a proven antibacterial agent that effectively inhibits the growth of *staphylococcus*.

❐ **Dosages:** To speed the healing of a lanced boil, apply a garlic poultice or fomentation to the affected area up to three times daily until it heals.

FUNGAL INFECTIONS

❒ **Symptoms:** Athlete's foot, jock itch, ringworm, yeast infections—these are all fungal infections caused by microscopic plants that become parasites on the skin. Called fungi, these small organisms cause localized itching, fluid-filled bumps, red or grayish scaly patches, and warmness at the site of infection.

❒ **How Garlic Can Help:** Garlic has traditionally been used to treat a wide range of fungal infections from athlete's foot to ringworm. Indeed, both clinical and human studies have shown that garlic has powerful fungal-fighting powers.

❒ **Dosages:** Apply a garlic poultice or fomentation to the affected area up to two times daily until the area heals. Or soak the infected area twice a day in warm water to which 5 grams of liquid extract, 5 grams of tincture, or 1 cup of garlic tea has been added.

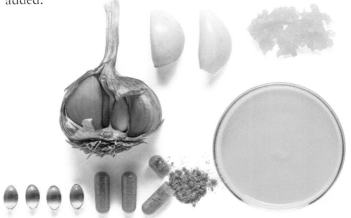

CONDITIONS AND DOSES

INSECT BITES AND STINGS

❒ **Symptoms:** Redness, inflammation, itching, and/or fever at the affected site. In some instances a localized infection may develop.

❒ **How Garlic Can Help:** Garlic stimulates the immune system to promote quicker healing. In instances where infection has set in, garlic's sulfur-containing compounds (ajoene, allicin, diallyl sulfide, diallyl disulfide, and diallyl trisulfide) increase the mobility of infection-fighting white blood cells and stimulate phagocytosis—the process in which white blood cells consume invading bacteria.

❒ **Dosages:** Apply a garlic poultice or fomentation to the affected area up to three times daily until the area heals. If an infection has set in, you can also take one 300-mg capsule of garlic three times daily before meals; or 5 grams of liquid extract or 5 grams of tincture three times daily before meals.

STOP THE STINGERS

Ouch! You've just been stung! Your next move is to remove the offending stinger. For years we've been told to scrape the stinger off the skin with a stiff object, such as a credit card. Yet according to a study published by the British medical journal, *Lancet*, if you act instantly, you are better off actually yanking the stinger from your skin rather than wasting precious seconds searching for a scraper to do the job. However, if the stinger has been in you a few seconds, go ahead and use your credit card. Hand-plucking it does carry the risk of sending more venom into your bloodstream–and if it's taken you awhile to act, you already have enough of the irritant under your skin without adding more.

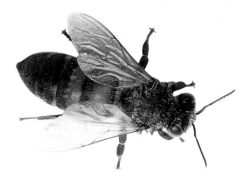

GROW IT YOURSELF

Known botanically as Allium sativum, garlic belongs to the wide-ranging lily family, a group that also includes leeks, onions, scallions, and shallots. A moderately-easy plant to grow, garlic is a perennial that displays attractive pink or purple blooms in spring and stalk-like leaves. If you'd like to try growing this eye-catching plant yourself, be aware that there are numerous varieties—some designed for northern or southern climates; some spicy and hot, others sweet and mellow; some with enormous bulbs, others more petite in size; some a purplish color, others a more traditional silvery white. Fortunately, all varieties offer both taste and a homegrown source of potent herbal medicine.

<u>GARLIC</u>

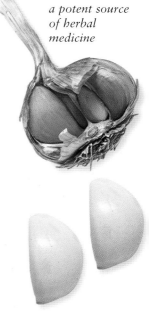

a potent source of herbal medicine

• **Size.** Up to 75 cm high.

• **Native Habitat.** Garlic's ancestral home is central Asia, which has long, cold winters, damp springs, and arid summers. However, there's barely a culture on earth that doesn't use garlic—both as a medicinal plant and a culinary seasoning. To accommodate everyone, garlic is now successfully cultivated in a variety of places, from Poland to Texas. Furthermore, there are dozens of garden varieties—all equally healthful—meaning there's a good chance that at least one garlic variety will grow in your family garden.

• **Cultivation.** Garlic prefers rich, loamy, well-drained soil. Start garlic in early fall so a mature root system can develop and take hold before winter frosts arrive. It is this strong root system that will be able to support the leafy "scapes" and pink or purple flowers that appear during the spring. Direct-seed individual cloves, planting each in an upright position about four to six inches apart and covering with an inch or two of dirt. While garlic likes slightly moist soil, it will rot if the ground becomes too wet. Bulbs are usually ready to harvest the following summer—from early July to mid-August—when foliage turns brown. To harvest, very gently pull each bulb up from the ground or carefully dig up each bulb.

• **Hint.** To store garlic, gently place bulbs in a dark, cool, well-ventilated location.

BEFORE GATHERING, ASK YOURSELF

✔ Is this plant endangered? If so, it may be illegal in your state to gather it.

✔ Do I need to take this herb from the wild or can I purchase it or grow it myself?

✔ Am I gathering for personal use only and not for commercial use? Note: Gathering wild plants for commercial use is illegal in many states.

✔ What part of the plant do I need? In the United States and Europe, garlic leaves are considered the medicinal portion of the plant. Leaves are best gathered in late summer when their active compounds are at their most concentrated.

✔ What will I be using this herb for and exactly how much of it do I need?

DO-IT-YOURSELF REMEDIES

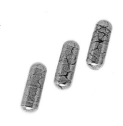

★ **Capsule:** Make your own herb supplements by purchasing animal or vegetable gelatin capsules at your local health food store and packing each individual capsule with 300 mg of dried, pulverized garlic or an equal amount of freshly minced garlic. **Standard dosage:** one 300-mg capsule three times daily.

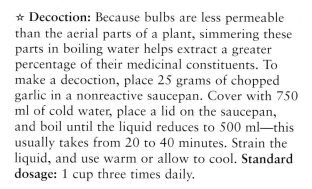

★ **Decoction:** Because bulbs are less permeable than the aerial parts of a plant, simmering these parts in boiling water helps extract a greater percentage of their medicinal constituents. To make a decoction, place 25 grams of chopped garlic in a nonreactive saucepan. Cover with 750 ml of cold water, place a lid on the saucepan, and boil until the liquid reduces to 500 ml—this usually takes from 20 to 40 minutes. Strain the liquid, and use warm or allow to cool. **Standard dosage:** 1 cup three times daily.

★ **Drying:** Peel and chop fresh garlic cloves into small pieces. Lay the chopped herb on trays in a dry, well-ventilated, nonsunny area of your home, or place in an extremely low oven, making sure air is continously circulating around the herbs. Or you can use a dehydrator. Drying will take between 7 and 14 days. When drying herbs either in a warm room or an oven, the temperature should be kept between 70° to 90° F. Store dried root in a dark, airtight, nonporous container.

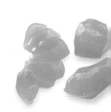

★ **Fomentation:** Fomentations are essentially gauze or surgical bandages that are soaked in freshly made herbal tea. The hot cloth is then laid directly on a bite, rash, or wound.

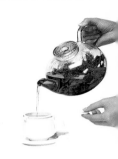

★ **Infused Oil Made With Fresh Leaves:** Infused oils boast the fat-soluble active principles of whatever medicinal plant or herb was used to make them. One way to create garlic oil is to tightly pack a clean jar to its top with fresh, crushed garlic cloves. Pour olive oil into the jar to cover the herb. Seal the jar tightly, and leave in a warm place for six to seven weeks. Shake it daily. When ready to use, strain the oil, and store in a dark, airtight container for up to two years. Can be ingested, added to foods, or used externally.

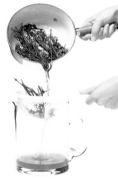

★ **Liquid Extract.** Also known as extract. To make garlic extract, macerate 300 to 500 grams of fresh garlic cloves. Place the herb in a jar and pour in 335 ml of vodka (37 proof or higher) and 165 ml of water. Place the lid on the jar and store in a dark area for four to eight weeks. Shake the mixture daily. When ready, strain the mixture, pressing all remaining liquid from the garlic cloves. Place liquid in a nonreactive saucepan and simmer over medium heat for 20 to 40 minutes until the liquid has been reduced by a third. This process burns off the alcohol, leaving the medicinal liquid behind. Allow liquid to cool and decant into several dropper bottles or a clean glass bottle. Will keep up to two years. **Standard dosage:** 5 ml three times daily.

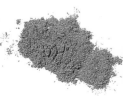

Do-It-Yourself Remedies

☆ **Ointment:** Also called a salve, herbal ointment is easy to make at home. To create your own garlic ointment, mix 1 to 2 parts beeswax or soft paraffin wax, 7 parts cocoa butter, and 3 parts pulverized dried garlic in a nonreactive saucepan. Cook the mixture for one to two hours on a low setting. Let cool, package in an airtight container, and apply up to three times daily.

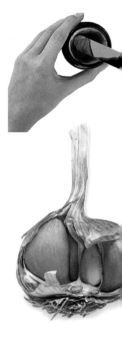

☆ **Poultice:** Fresh herbs can be applied directly to the skin when fashioned into a poultice. To make a garlic poultice, chop fresh cloves. Boil in a small amount of water for 5 minutes (or use a microwave). Squeeze out any excess liquid from the boiled herb (reserve liquid). Lay the garlic directly on the skin and cover with a warm moist towel. Leave in place for up to 30 minutes. The reserved liquid can be rewarmed and used to reheat the towel.

☆ **Syrup:** Garlic has a pronounced taste that may not be palatable to some individuals. Syrup delivers the herb's medicinal benefits in an easy-to-swallow (and throat-soothing) base. To make, mix 7 parts garlic tea or decoction in a nonreactive saucepan with 10 parts sugar. Cook the mixture over low heat until it has formed a thick, syrupy consistency. For coughs and sore

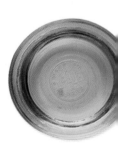

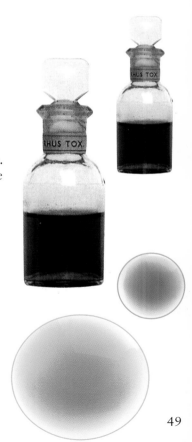

throats, take 1 or 2 tablespoons up to four times daily.

☆ **Tea:** Also known as an infusion, tea is an easy and common way to ingest an herb. To make garlic tea, steep 1 garlic clove for five minutes in 1 cup of boiling water. You may add fructose, sugar, or honey to sweeten. **Standard dosage:** 1 cup of tea three times daily.

☆ **Tinctures:** Though they are not as potent as liquid extracts, tinctures are minimally processed, making them a favorite remedy among many herbalists. To make your own garlic tincture, place 300 to 500 grams of fresh, crushed garlic cloves in a large jar and cover with 500 ml of vodka (37 proof or higher). Place the lid on the jar and store in a dark area for four to six weeks. Shake the bottle daily. When ready to use, strain the mixture, pressing all remaining liquid from the garlic cloves. Decant into several dropper bottles or a clean glass bottle. Will keep for up to two years. Shake before using. **Standard dosage:** 5 ml three times daily.

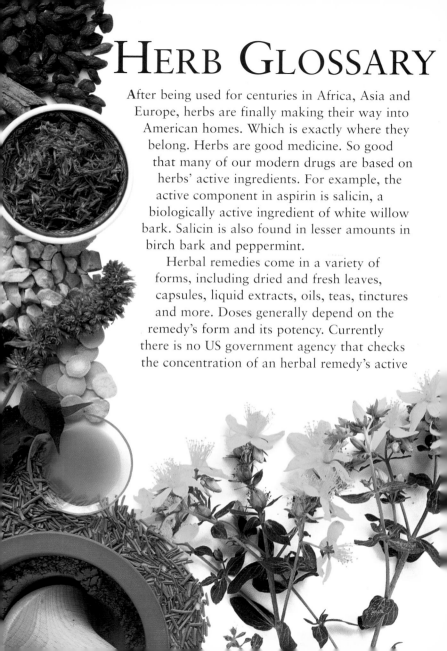

HERB GLOSSARY

After being used for centuries in Africa, Asia and Europe, herbs are finally making their way into American homes. Which is exactly where they belong. Herbs are good medicine. So good that many of our modern drugs are based on herbs' active ingredients. For example, the active component in aspirin is salicin, a biologically active ingredient of white willow bark. Salicin is also found in lesser amounts in birch bark and peppermint.

Herbal remedies come in a variety of forms, including dried and fresh leaves, capsules, liquid extracts, oils, teas, tinctures and more. Doses generally depend on the remedy's form and its potency. Currently there is no US government agency that checks the concentration of an herbal remedy's active

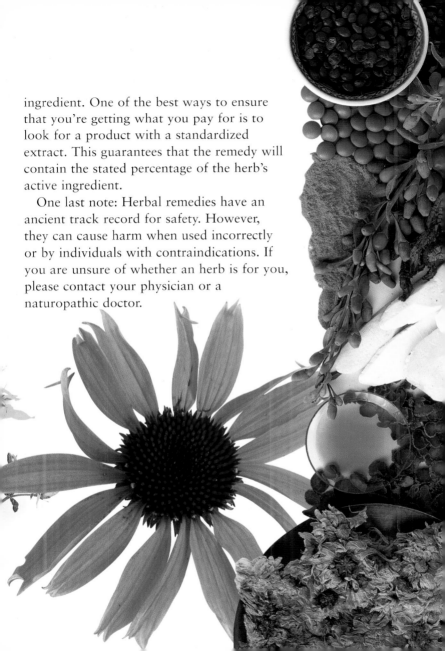

ingredient. One of the best ways to ensure that you're getting what you pay for is to look for a product with a standardized extract. This guarantees that the remedy will contain the stated percentage of the herb's active ingredient.

One last note: Herbal remedies have an ancient track record for safety. However, they can cause harm when used incorrectly or by individuals with contraindications. If you are unsure of whether an herb is for you, please contact your physician or a naturopathic doctor.

ALOE

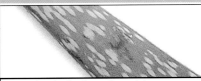

Properties: Analgesic, antibacterial, antifungal, anti-inflammatory, anti-itch, antiseptic, circulatory stimulant, digestive aid, immune-system stimulant, laxative.
Target Ailments: Acne, bruises, burns, constipation, cuts, insect bites, digestive disorders, rashes, ulcers, wounds.
Available Forms: Capsule, fresh leaves, gel, juice, liquid extract.
Possible Side Effects: When taken internally, aloe can cause severe cramping in some individuals.
Precautions: Pregnant women should not ingest aloe; It can stimulate uterine contractions.

CALENDULA

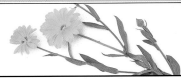

Properties: Antibacterial, anti-inflammatory, antiseptic, antispasmodic, promotes sweating, sedative.
Target Ailments: Burns, cuts, fungal infections, gallbladder conditions, hepatitis, indigestion, irregular menstruation, insect bites, menstrual cramps, mouth sores, skin rashes, ulcers, wounds.
Available Forms: Capsule, dried herb, fresh herb, liquid extract, lotion, oil, ointment, tincture.
Possible Side Effects: None expected.
Precautions: Calendula is related to ragweed. Individuals allergic to ragweed should consult a physician before using calendula.

ASTRAGALUS

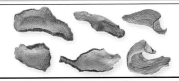

Properties: Antibacterial, anti-inflammatory, antioxidant, antiviral, diuretic, immune-system stimulant.
Target Ailments: Cancer, colds, appetite loss, diarrhea, fatigue, flu, heart conditions, HIV, viral infections.
Available Forms: Capsule, dried herb, fresh herb, liquid extract, tea, tincture.
Possible Side Effects: None expected.
Precautions: Astragalus should be used as a companion therapy to—not a replacement for—traditional cancer and HIV therapies.

CHAMOMILE

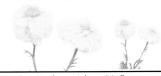

Properties: Antibacterial, anti-inflammatory, antiseptic, antispasmodic, carminative, digestive aid, fever reducer, sedative.
Target Ailments: Gingivitis, hemorrhoids, insomnia, indigestion, intestinal gas, menstrual cramps, nausea, nervousness, stomachaches, sunburns, tension, ulcers, varicose veins.
Available Forms: Capsule, dried herb, fresh herb, liquid extract, lotion, oil, tea, tincture.
Possible Side Effects: None expected.
Precautions: Because chamomile is related to ragweed, individuals with ragweed allergies should consult a physician before using chamomile.

DONG QUAI

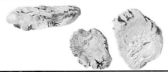

Properties: Antiallergenic, antispasmodic, diuretic, mild laxative, muscle relaxant, vasodilator.
Target Ailments: Abscesses, blurred vision, heart palpitations, irregular menstruation, light-headedness, menstrual pain, pallor, poor circulation.
Available Forms: Capsule, dried herb, liquid extract, tincture.
Possible Side Effects: Can cause photosensitivity in some individuals.
Precautions: Dong quai has abortive abilities; Do not take while pregnant.

FEVERFEW

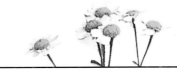

Properties: Anti-inflammatory, fever reducer.
Target Ailments: Arthritis, asthma, dermatitis, menstrual pain, migraines.
Available Forms: Capsule, dried herb, fresh herb, liquid extract, tincture.
Possible Side Effects: Some individuals experience "withdrawal" symptoms after taking feverfew, including fatigue and nervousness.
Precautions: Because it is related to ragweed, individuals with ragweed allergies should consult a physician before using feverfew.

ECHINACEA

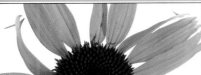

Properties: Antiallergenic, antibacterial, antiseptic, antimicrobial, antiviral, carminative, lymphatic tonic.
Target Ailments: Abscesses, acne, bladder infections, blood poisoning, burns, colds, eczema, food poisoning, flu, insect bites, kidney infections, mononucleosis, respiratory infections, sore throats.
Available Forms: Capsule, dried herb, liquid extract, tea, tincture.
Possible Side Effects: High doses can cause dizziness and nausea.
Precautions: Do not take echinacea for more than four weeks in a row.

GARLIC

Properties: Antibacterial, anticoagulant, antifungal, anti-inflammatory, antiviral, cholesterol reducer, digestive aid, immune-system stimulant, worm-fighting.
Target Ailments: Arteriosclerosis, arthritis, bladder infections, colds, digestive upset, flu, heart conditions, high blood pressure, high blood cholesterol, viral infections.
Available Forms: Capsule, fresh cloves, liquid extract, oil, tincture.
Possible Side Effects: Can cause upset stomach.
Precautions: While garlic is safe taken in culinary doses, individuals on anticoagulant medications should consult their doctors before supplementing their diet with garlic.

GINGER

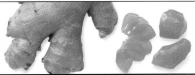

Properties: Antibacterial, anticoagulant, antinausea, antispasmodic, antiviral, carminative, digestive aid, expectorant, immune-system stimulant, muscle relaxant.
Target Ailments: Burns, colds, flu, high blood pressure, high cholesterol, liver conditions, intestinal gas, menstrual cramps, motion sickness, nausea, stomachaches.
Available Forms: Capsule, dried root, tea.
Possible Side Effects: Heartburn.
Precautions: While ginger is safe in culinary doses, individuals who suffer from a blood-clotting disorder or are on anticoagulant medication should consult a physician before supplementing their diet with the herb.

GINSENG

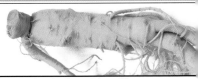

Properties: Antibacterial, antidepressant, immune-system stimulant, stimulant.
Target Ailments: Colds, depression, fatigue, flu, impaired immune system, respiratory conditions, stress.
Available Forms: Capsule, dried root, fresh root, liquid extract, tincture, tea.
Possible Side Effects: Large doses of ginseng can cause breast soreness, headaches or skin rashes in some individuals.
Precautions: Ginseng can aggravate existing heart palpitations or high blood pressure.

GINKGO BILOBA

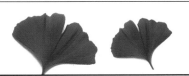

Properties: Antibacterial, anti-inflammatory, antioxidant, circulatory stimulant, vasodilator.
Target Ailments: Clotting disorders, dementia, depression, headaches, hearing loss, Raynaud's syndrome, tinnitus, vascular diseases, vertigo.
Available Forms: Capsule, dry herb, liquid extract, tincture, tea.
Possible Side Effects: Diarrhea, irritability, nausea, restlessness.
Precautions: Do not use ginkgo biloba if you have a blood-clotting disorder like hemophilia or are taking anticoagulant medications.

GOLDENSEAL

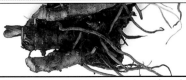

Properties: Antacid, antibacterial, antifungal, anti-inflammatory, antiseptic, astringent, digestive aid, stimulant.
Target Ailments: Canker sores, contact dermatitis, diarrhea, eczema, food poisoning.
Available Forms: Capsule, dry herb, liquid extract, tincture.
Possible Side Effects: In high doses, goldenseal can cause diarrhea and nausea and can irritate the skin, mouth and throat.
Precautions: Because of its high cost, many manufacturers adulterate preparations with less costly herbs, such as barberry, yellow dock or bloodroot, some of which can cause unwanted reactions when taken in high doses.

KAVA

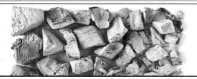

Properties: Antidepressant, antispasmodic, aphrodisiac, diuretic, muscle relaxant, sedative.
Target Ailments: Anxiety, colds, depression, menstrual conditions, muscle cramps, respiratory tract conditions, stress.
Available Forms: Capsule, dried herb, liquid extract, tea, tincture.
Possible Side Effects: Allergic skin reactions, muscle weakness, red eyes, sleepiness.
Precautions: In high doses, kava can impair motor reflexes and cause breathing problems.

MILK THISTLE

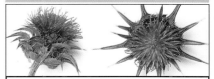

Properties: Anti-inflammatory, antioxidant, digestive aid, immune-system stimulant.
Target Ailments: inflammation of the gallbladder duct, hepatitis, liver conditions, poisoning from ingestion of the death cup mushroom, psoriasis.
Available Forms: Capsule, dried herb, fresh herb, powder, tea, tincture.
Possible Side Effects: Milk thistle can cause mild diarrhea when taken in large doses.
Precautions: If you think you have a liver disorder, seek medical advice before taking this herb.

LAVENDER

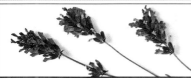

Properties: Antibacterial, antidepressant, antiseptic, antispasmodic, carminative, circulatory stimulant, digestive aid, diuretic, sedative.
Target Ailments: Anxiety, depression, headache, insomnia, intestinal gas, nausea, tension.
Available Forms: Capsule, dried herb, fresh herb, oil, tincture.
Possible Side Effects: Lavender products can cause skin irritation in sensitive individuals.
Precautions: Lavender oil is poisonous when ingested internally.

PARSLEY

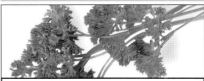

Properties: Antiseptic, antispasmodic, digestive aid, diuretic, laxative, muscle relaxant.
Target Ailments: Colds, congestion, fever, flu, indigestion, irregular menstruation, premenstrual syndrome, stimulating the production of breast milk, stomachaches.
Available Forms: Capsule, dried herb, fresh herb, liquid extract, oil, tea, tincture.
Possible Side Effects: Can cause photosensitivity in some individuals.
Precautions: Parsley should not be ingested in large amounts or used externally during pregnancy; it contains compounds that may stimulate uterine muscles and possibly cause miscarriage.

PEPPERMINT

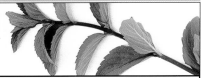

Properties: Antacid, antibacterial, antidepressant, antispasmodic, carminatve, expectorant, muscle relaxant, promotes sweating.
Target Ailments: Anxiety, colds, fever, flu, insomnia, intestinal gas, itching, migraines, morning sickness, motion sickness, nausea.
Available Forms: Capsule, dried herb, fresh herb, lozenge, oil, ointment, tea, tincture.
Possible Side Effects: When applied externally, peppermint products can cause skin reactions in sensitive individuals.
Precautions: If you have a hiatal hernia, talk to your doctor before using peppermint products externally or internally; the oil in the plant can exacerbate symptoms.

SAGE

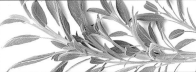

Properties: Antiseptic, anti-inflammatory, antioxidant, antispasmodic, astringent, bile stimulant, carminative, reduces perspiration.
Target Ailments: Excess intestinal gas, insect bites, menopausal night sweats, poor circulation, reduces milk flow at weaning, sore throat, stomachaches, mouth ulcers.
Available Forms: Capsule, dried herb, fresh herb, liquid extract, oil, tincture.
Possible Side Effects: Sage tea may cause inflammation of the lips and/or tongue in some individuals.
Precautions: Do not ingest pure sage oil; it is toxic when taken internally.

ROSEMARY

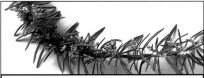

Properties: Antibacterial, antidepressant, anti-inflammatory, antiseptic, carminative, circultory stimulant.
Target Ailments: Bad breath, dandruff, depression, eczema, headaches, indigestion, joint inflammation, mouth and throat infections, muscle pain, psoriasis, rheumatoid arthritis.
Available Forms: Dried herb, fresh herb, ingestible rosemary-flavored oil, oil, ointment, tea, tincture.
Possible Side Effects: Rosemary oil can cause skin inflammation and/or dermatitis.
Precautions: Do not mistake regular rosemary oil for ingestible rosemary-flavored oil.

SAW PALMETTO

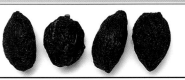

Properties: Antiallergenic, anti-inflammatory, diuretic, immune-boosting.
Target Ailments: Asthma, benign prostatic hyperplasia, bronchitis, colds, cystitis, impotence, male infertility, nasal congestion, sinus conditions, sore throats.
Available Forms: Capsule, dried herb, fresh herb, liquid extract, oil, tea, tincture.
Possible Side Effects: Can cause diarrhea if taken in large doses.
Precautions: Due to its hormonal actions, saw palmetto may interact negatively with prostate medicines or hormonal treatments such as estrogen replacement therapy, possibly canceling out their effectiveness.

ST. JOHN'S WORT

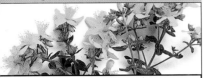

Properties: Analgesic, antibacterial, anti-depressant, anti-inflammatory, antiviral, astringent.
Target Ailments: Attention deficit disorder, anxiety, bacterial infections, burns, carpal tunnel syndrome, depression, HIV, menopause.
Available Forms: Capsule, dried herb, liquid extract, oil, ointment, tea, tincture.
Possible Side Effects: Gastrointestinal upset, headaches, photosensitivity, stiff neck.
Precautions: Avoid foods containing the amino acid tyramine when taking St. John's wort; the interaction of the two can cause an increase in blood pressure. Foods with tyramine include beer, coffee, wine, chocolate and fava beans.

WILD YAM

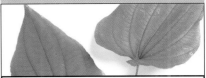

Properties: Analgesic, anti-inflammatory, antispasmodic, expectorant, muscle relaxant, promotes sweating.
Target Ailments: Menopause, menstrual cramps, morning sickness, nausea, rheumatoid arthritis, urinary tract infections.
Available Forms: Capsule, cream, dried root, liquid extract, oil, powder, tincture.
Possible Side Effects: Can cause vomiting in large doses.
Precautions: Individuals who are suffering from a hormone-sensitive cancer, such as breast or uterine cancer, should avoid wild yam. Some experts believe that the herb can encourage the growth of cancer cells.

VALERIAN

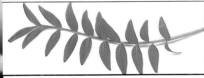

Properties: Analgesic, antibacterial, antispasmodic, carminative, reduces blood pressure, sedative, tranquilizer.
Target Ailments: Brachial spasm, high blood pressure, insomnia, palpitations, menstrual pain, migraines, muscle cramps, nervousness, tension headaches, wounds.
Available Forms: Capsules, dried herb, liquid extract, oil, teas, tincture.
Possible Side Effects: Headaches with prolonged use.
Precautions: Do not take with other sedatives, including alcohol. Do not drive or operate machinery after taking valerian.

YARROW

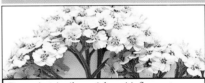

Properties: Antibacterial, anti-inflammatory, antispasmodic, blood coagulator, bile stimulating, immune-system stimulant, promotes sweating, sedative.
Target Ailments: Anxiety, colds and flu, cystitis, digestive disorders, menstrual cramps, minor wounds, nosebleeds, poor circulation, skin rashes.
Available Forms: Dried herb, capsule, liquid extract, oil, tea, tincture.
Possible Side Effects: Diarrhea, skin rash.
Precautions: Yarrow is related to ragweed and can cause an allergic reaction in individuals with ragweed allergies. Do not take if pregnant; it can induce miscarriage.

Herbal Terms

You're thumbing through the latest herbal therapy book when you run smack into the word "emmenagogue." Or perhaps you get tangled on "oxytocic." For anyone who's ever been stopped by an unfamiliar alternative medical term, we offer the following list:

Adaptogenic: Increases resistance and resilience to stress. Supports adrenal gland functioning.

Alterative: Blood purifier that improves the condition of the blood, improves digestion, and increases the appetite. Used to treat conditions arising from or causing toxicity.

Analgesic: Herb that relieves pain either by relaxing muscles or reducing pain signals to the brain.

Anthelmintic: Destroys or expels intestinal worms.

Antacid: Neutralizes excess stomach and intestinal acids.

Antiallergenic: Inactivates allergenic substances in the body.

Antibacterial/Antibiotic: Helps the body fight off harmful bacteria.

Antidepressant: Helps maintain emotional stability.

Anticatarrhal: Eliminates or counteracts the formation of mucus.

Anticoagulant: Thins blood and helps prevent blood clots.

Antifungal: Kills infection-causing fungi.

Anti-inflammatory: Reduces swelling of the tissues.

Anti-itch: Deadens itching sensations.

Antimicrobial: Kills a wide range of harmful bacteria, fungi, and viruses.

Antioxidant: Fights harmful oxidation.

Antipyretic/Fever Reducer: Reduces or prevents fever.

Antiseptic: External application prevents bacterial growth on skin.

Antispasmodic: Prevents or relaxes muscle tension.

Antiviral: Helps the body fight invading viruses.

Astringent: Has a constricting or binding effect. Commonly used to treat hemorrhages, secretions and diarrhea.

Blood Coagulant: Thickens blood and aids in clotting.

Carminative: Relieves gas.

Cholagogue: Encourages the flow of bile into the small intestine.

Circulatory Stimulant: Promotes even and efficient blood circulation.

Demulcent: Soothing substance, usually mucilage, taken internally to protect injured or inflamed tissues.

Diaphoretic: Induces sweating.

Diuretic: Increases urine flow.

Emetic: Induces vomiting.

Emmenagogue: Promotes menstruation.

Emollient: Softens, soothes and protects skin.

Expectorant: Assists in expelling mucus from the lungs and throat.

Galactogogue: Increases the secretion of breast milk.

Hemostatic: Stops hemorrhaging and encourages blood coagulation.

Hepatic: Tones and strengthens the liver.

Hypotensive: Lowers abnormally elevated blood pressure.

Immune-System Stimulant: Strengthens immune system so the body can fight off invading organisms.

Laxative: Promotes bowel movements.

Lithotriptic: Helps dissolve urinary and biliary stones.

Muscle Relaxant: Loosens tight muscles and reduces muscle cramping.

Nervine: Calms tension.

Oxytocic: Stimulates uterine contractions.

Rubefacient: Increases blood flow at the surface of the skin.

Sedative: Quiets the nervous system.

Sialagogue/Digestive Aid: Promotes the flow of saliva.

Stimulant: Increases the body's energy.

Tonic: Promotes the functions of body systems.

Vasoconstrictor: Constricts blood vessels, limiting the amount of blood flowing to a particular area.

Vasodilator: Dilates blood vessels, helping to promote blood flow.

Vulnerary: Encourages wound healing by promoting cell growth and repair.

HERBAL ORGANIZATIONS

Where to go for more information:

American Botanical Council
P.O. Box 201660
Austin, TX 78720
512-331-8868
www.herbalgram.org

The American Herbalist Guild
P.O. Box 746555
Arvada, CO 80006
303-423-8800

American Herbalists Guild
Box 1683
Soquel, CA 95073
408-464-2441

Herb Research Foundation
1007 Pearl Street, Suite 200
Boulder, CO 80302
303-449-2265
www.herbs.org

**National Accupuncture and
Oriental Medicine Alliance**
14637 Starr Road SE
Olalla, WA 98359
206-851-6896

**National Institutes of Health
Office of Alternative Medicine**
9000 Rockville Pike
Building 31, Room 5B-37
Mailstop 2182
Bethesda, MD 20892
301-402-2466

The Herb Society of America
9019 Kirtland-Chardon Road
Kirtland, OH 44094
216-256-0514

American College of Sports Medicine
P.O. Box 1440
Indianapolis, IN 46206
317-637-9200

American Heart Association
7272 Greenville Avenue
Dallas, TX 75231
214-373-6300

National Health Information Center
P.O. Box 1133
Washington, DC 20013
800-336-4797

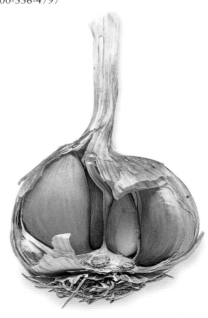

GROWING HERBS

Interested in cultivating herbs yourself?
These sources can supply roots, plants, and/or seeds.

Catoctin Mountain Botanicals
P.O. Box 454
Jefferson, MD 21755
301-473-4351

Companion Plants
7247 N. Coolville Ridge Rd.
Athens, OH 45701
614-593-3092
E-mail: complants@frognet.net

Dry Fork Herb Gardens
R.R.#1 Box 21
Rockport, IL
217-437-5281

Ecofriendly Farms
15488 Barn Rock Rd.
Mendota, VA 24270
540-466-8689

Goodwin Creek Gardens
P.O. Box 83
Williams, OR 97544
541-846-7357

Herbal Exchange
P.O. Box 429
9160 Lentz Rd.
Frazeysburg, OH 43822
614-828-9968

Horizon Herbs
P.O. Box 69
Williams, OR 97544
541-846-6233
www.chatlink.com/~herbseed
E-mail: herbseed@chatlink.com

Johnny's Seeds
Rt. 1 Box 2580
Foss Hill Rd.
Albion, ME 04910
207-437-9294
www.johnnyseeds.com

Mountain Traditions
H.C. 68, Box 193
Big Creek, KY 40914
606-598-6904

Nature's Cathedral
Rt. 1 Box 120
Blairstown, IA 52209
319-454-6959

Prairie Moon Nursery
Rt. 3, Box 163
Winona, MN 55987
507-452-1362

Wilcox Natural Products
P.O. Box 391
755 George Wilson Rd.
Boone, NC 28607
828-264-3615
www.goldenseal.com

Wild Wonderful Farm, Inc.
P.O. Box 256
Franklin, W'
212-736-14€

Natural Care

INDEX

——— A ———

acne, 38
ajoene, 7, 42
alcohol, 18, 29
alliin and allicin, 7, 16, 17, 24, 32, 33, 42
Allium sativum, 53
common names for, 7
defense mechanism of, 33
how to grow, 44–45
allopathic medicine, 8, 10. See also Antibiotics
allyl propyl disulfide, 32
aloe, 52
alternative medicine, 4–5, 6, 8. See also
Chinese medicine
antibiotic properties, 6, 27, 29, 33, 38
antibiotics, 8
anticancer properties, 7, 22–23
antifungal properties, 33, 41
antihelmintic properties, 6, 36–37
antioxidant properties, 16, 33
antiviral properties, 6, 26, 27, 29, 30, 33
astragalus, 52
astringent properties, 6, 38
athlete's foot, 41
Ayurvedic medicine, 4, 8

——— B ———

blood cholesterol, high, 18
blood pressure, 20
blood sugar, 7, 13, 32
blood-thinning properties, 7, 13, 16, 18, 20
boils, 40
breath, "garlic," 21
bronchitis, acute, 24
buying tips, 17

——— C ———

calendula, 52
cancer, 7, 22–23
capsules, 14, 46
cardiovascular conditions, 7, 16–21
carminatives, 7
chamomile, 52
chemical exposure, limitation of, 19
Chinese medicine, 4
cholesterol, high blood levels, 18
colds, 24, 26–27, 29
Commission E of Germany, 8
contraindications. See Safety issues
coronary artery disease, 7, 16–17, 32
cultivation, 45

——— D ———

decoction, 46

definitions, 58–59
diabetes, 32–33
diallyl sulfides, 7, 16, 17, 22, 29, 42
dietary factors, 16, 37
digestives, 7
diuretics, 7
do-it-yourself remedies, 46
dong quai, 53
dosage, 17. See also individual conditions
dried herbs, 14, 46

——— E ———

echinacea, 53
environmental exposure to toxins, 19
Epstein-Barr virus, 30
essential oil, 14
exercise, 25
expectorants, 7
extract. See Liquid extract

——— F ———

fatigue, 34
feverfew, 53
fiber, importance of, 37
fomentation, 47
fresh herbs, 14, 47
fungal infections, 33, 41

——— G ———

garlic. See Allium sativum
"garlic breath," 21
ginger, 54
ginkgo biloba, 54
ginseng, 54
glossaries
for formats for herbal medicines, 14–15, 46–49
of herbs, 50–57
glucosinolates, 7
goldenseal, 54
growth characteristics, 44

——— H ———

habitat, 44
harvesting, 45
herbalism, Western, 4–5, 6, 22
herbal terms, 58–59
herbs
dried, 14, 46
fresh, 14, 47
glossary of, 50–57
herpes virus, 30
historical usage, 4–5, 6, 22, 26, 34, 36
homeopathy, 8
hormones, stress and, 35

hypertension, 20
hypoglycemia, 13

—————— I ——————
immune system, 6, 24, 25, 26, 27, 29, 30, 35, 40, 42
influenza, 24, 27, 28, 29
infused oil, 15, 47
infusion. See Tea
insect bites and stings, 42–43
intestinal parasites, 6, 36–37

—————— J ——————
jock itch, 41
juices, 14

—————— K ——————
kava, 55

—————— L ——————
lavender, 55
liquid extract, 14, 46

—————— M ——————
mechanisms of action, 7, 17, 29. See also individual conditions
medicinal properties, 6–7
S-methyl-L-cysteine sulfoxide, 7
milk thistle, 55
mononucleosis, 30

—————— N ——————
names, common, 7
National Formulary, 6
Native American medicine, 5

—————— O ——————
oils. See Essential oil; Infused oil
ointment, 15, 48
organic foods, 31
organizations, 60–61

—————— P ——————
pancreas, function of the, 32
parasites, intestinal, 6, 36–37
parsley, 55
peppermint, 56
physical activity, 25
poultices, 48

—————— Q ——————
questions to ask yourself, 9, 11, 45

—————— R ——————
radiation therapy, 23

remedies, do-it-yourself, 46
research, 8, 23, 34, 35
resources, 60–61
ringworm, 41
rosemary, 56

—————— S ——————
safety issues, 9, 11, 13
sage, 56
St. John's wort, 57
saw palmetto, 56
seed suppliers, 61
selenium, 7, 22
side effects, 12, 38
skin conditions, 13, 38–43
skin irritation, 13, 39
smoking, 16, 18, 29
sore throat, 24, 27, 28, 29
stings, insect, 42–43
storage tips, 45
stress, 16, 35
supplies, where to order, 61
surgery, caution with, 13
susceptibility to infections, 29. See also Immune system
syrups, 15, 48–49

—————— T ——————
taxonomy, 7
tea, 15, 24, 27, 28, 29, 49
terms, 58–59
tinctures, 15, 49
traditional medicine, 4–5, 8. See also Chinese medicine

—————— U ——————
United States Pharmacopoeia, 6

—————— V ——————
valerian, 57
vegetarian diet, 18

—————— W ——————
wild yam, 57

—————— Y ——————
yarrow, 57
yeast infection, 41

ABOUT THE AUTHOR

Stephanie Pedersen is a writer and editor who specializes in the area of health. Her articles have appeared in numerous publications, including *American Woman, Sassy, Teen, Weight Watchers* and *Woman's World.* She has also co-written *What Your Cat is Trying to Tell You: A Head-to-Tail Guide to Your Cat's Symptoms and Their Solutions* and *What Your Dog is Trying to Tell You: A Head-to-Tail Guide to Your Dog's Symptoms and Their Solutions,* both published by St. Martin's Press. She currently resides in New York City.

Picture Credits: Steve Gorton, David Murray, Dave King, Martin Norris, Philip Gatward, Andy Crawford, Philip Dowell, Clive Streeter, Peter Chadwick, Tim Ridley, Andrew Whittack, Martin Cameron

DORLING KINDERSLEY PUBLISHING, INC.
www.dk.com

Published in the United States by
Dorling Kindersley Publishing, Inc.
95 Madison Avenue • New York, New York 10016

Editorial Director: LaVonne Carlson
Editors: Nancy Burke, Barbara Minton, Connie Robinson
Designer: Carol Wells
Cover Designer: Gus Yoo

Pedersen, Stephanie.
    Garlic : immunity booster and inflammation reducer / by Stephanie Pedersen.
    p. cm. -- (Natural care library)
    Includes index.
    ISBN 0-7894-5192-1 (pbk. : alk. paper)
    1. Garlic--Therapeutic use. I. Title. II. Series.
RM666.G15P43 2000
615'. 32433--dc21
99-43068

First American Edition 1999   2 4 6 8 10 9 7 5 3